The Mitochondrial Miracle

Reclaiming Your Health and Vitality

Dr. Nikolai J. Graham

Disclaimer

This book's content is intended solely for educational purposes and should not be construed as medical advice. It is not intended to diagnose or serve as a substitute for professional medical monitoring. Before using any information offered, it is advised to speak with a healthcare provider about any medical condition.

Neither the publisher nor the author shall be liable for any harm purportedly caused by any information in this book.

Table of Contents

Chapter One

Understanding Mitochondria

The Mitochondrial Miracle: Regaining Your Health and Vitality: An Understanding of Mitochondria

Inside cells, mitochondria are tiny, bean-shaped organelles that are essential for energy production. Their production of adenosine triphosphate (ATP), which cells use as fuel, has earned them the moniker "powerhouses" of the cell. According to recent studies, mitochondria play a far more intricate role in cellular function than previously thought, including signaling, regulation, and even cell formation and function control.

According to the mitochondrial theory of aging, cellular aging and a reduction in function are caused by the buildup of damaged mitochondria and reactive oxygen species

(ROS) in cells. Age-related illnesses and disorders may arise because mitochondrial DNA (mtDNA) mutates more frequently than nuclear DNA. Contradictory data from recent research, however, points to a more nuanced understanding of the role of mitochondria in aging.

The significance of mitochondria for general health and wellbeing will be explained in this book "The Mitochondrial Miracle: Reclaiming Your Health and Vitality." The following subjects will be covered in the book:

1. The function of mitochondria in cells: Energy generation, the metabolism of lipids and amino acids, and the control of apoptosis all depend on mitochondria. Additionally, they are involved in regulatory and signaling processes that govern cell growth and function.

2. Mitochondrial dynamics: Within cells, mitochondria undergo continuous morphological changes as a result of cycles of fusion and fission, generating extremely dynamic, transient tubular networks. They are

able to react to external stimuli and adjust to shifting cellular requirements thanks to their dynamic behavior.

3. Mitochondrial DNA and Aging: According to the mitochondrial theory of aging, cellular function declines and age-related illnesses emerge as a result of mtDNA mutations and the buildup of ROS-induced damage. Recent research, however, has called into question this notion and suggests that the role of mitochondria in aging is more nuanced than previously believed.

4. Strategies for regaining health and vitality: This book will give it's audience doable suggestions for enhancing their mitochondrial health, such as dietary adjustments, physical activity, and lifestyle adjustments. These tactics are meant to assist people in leading more vital, happier, and healthier lives.

"The Mitochondrial Miracle: Reclaiming Your Health and Vitality" will provide it's audience with a thorough grasp of how important mitochondria are to general health and wellbeing, in addition to helpful guidance on how to enhance their own mitochondrial vitality.

- The role of mitochondria in health and vitality

An essential part of every cell's operation and general well-being is the mitochondria. They are in charge of generating energy and are necessary for metabolism, vigor, and other physiological functions. Energy levels, concentration, and the capacity to maintain high levels of activity without becoming fatigued are all directly impacted by the quantity of healthy mitochondria in the body. Aging and the prevention of many diseases, including cancer, heart disease, and cognitive decline, are intimately related to mitochondrial health. Good nutrition, regular exercise, and enough sleep all support the upkeep of healthy mitochondria. Monitoring variables like membrane potential, shape, and the buildup of reactive oxygen species (ROS) is part of evaluating the health of the mitochondria. Numerous methods are used to assess mitochondrial health at the cellular level, such as high-content imaging systems and fluorescent dyes. Furthermore, it has been demonstrated that micronutrients like CoQ10 and B vitamins assist mitochondrial metabolism and energy production. For the purpose of fostering general health, good aging, and illness prevention, it is imperative to nourish and promote the mitochondria.

Mitochondria have a complex function in different areas of health and vitality, and maintaining them is essential for overall health and vitality. The search results shed light on the significance of mitochondrial health, the variables that affect it, and the techniques employed to measure it.

The human body is a marvel of complex biological systems, with the mitochondria serving as the powerhouse that maintains cellular health. The significant significance of these cellular powerhouses in maintaining health and vitality is examined in "The Mitochondrial Miracle," which offers an engrossing voyage into the science of energy production and general well-being.

Understanding Mitochondrial Function: Powerhouses of the Cell.

This explores the basic workings of mitochondria, highlighting their vital function in producing adenosine triphosphate (ATP), the energy unit of cells. The intriguing symbiotic link between mitochondria and the cell, highlighting the effects of effective energy production on a number of physiological functions.

Mitochondria and Cellular Resilience.

This explores the role mitochondria play in the body's resilience and reveals the complex web of antioxidant defenses and repair systems. It talks about how healthy mitochondria are essential for maintaining cellular viability and longevity by shielding cells from oxidative stress in addition to producing energy.

The Relationship Between Mitochondrial Health.

The extensive effects of mitochondrial health on general wellbeing are examined in this section. Readers learn about the enormous impact of healthy, functional mitochondria on preserving vibrant health and vitality, ranging from immune system support to hormonal balance.

Lifestyle and Dietary Practices for Mitochondrial Health

Given that lifestyle and diet have a significant impact on mitochondrial health, this chapter offers helpful advice on creating an environment that is conducive to mitochondrial health. With practical advice on everything from the advantages of particular diets to the importance of consistent exercise, readers may improve their mitochondrial miracle.

Managing the Sands of Time: Mitochondria and Aging.

This explores the aging process and provides insights on how mitochondrial activity varies with age and how to promote healthy aging. Understanding how to slow down aging-related deterioration and use the mitochondrial miracle to maintain energy is imparted to readers.

Unlocking the Mitochondrial Miracle: Future Perspectives and Therapeutic Strategies.

This will examine novel studies and treatment modalities meant to maximize mitochondrial performance. Readers are encouraged to imagine a future in which the mitochondrial marvel continues to develop, opening up new possibilities for health and vitality, from cutting-edge technologies to creative treatments.

To sum up, "The Mitochondrial Miracle" is a knowledge-aiding guide that leads individuals through the complex world of mitochondria and their exceptional function in promoting health and vitality. Through this exploration, people are encouraged to embrace the power within their cells and set out on a journey to fully realize the miracle of the mitochondria.

- Basic science of mitochondria and energy production

The creation of energy and general health and vigor depend on mitochondria, which are critical organelles. They are in charge of using the energy released by food oxidation to produce adenosine triphosphate (ATP) through oxidative phosphorylation. For the majority of biochemical and physiological functions, including growth, mobility, and equilibrium, ATP is the main energy source. The preservation of robust mitochondria is essential for maintaining energy levels, concentration, and the body's capacity to do intense physical activity without feeling tired. Beyond generating energy, mitochondria are also engaged in a number of other functions, such as iron metabolism and cellular process regulation.

The fundamental science of mitochondria and energy generation is closely related to general well-being. Stress reduction, exercise, sleep patterns, and a balanced diet are all important for mitochondrial health. Micronutrients that assist mitochondrial metabolism and energy production include CoQ10 and B vitamins In addition, sustaining the optimal operation of mitochondria requires proper feeding and maintenance, which includes eating a diet rich in whole foods that is well-balanced.

Monitoring variables like membrane potential, shape, and the buildup of reactive oxygen species (ROS) is part of evaluating the health of the mitochondria. Fluorescent dyes and high-content imaging techniques are used to assess mitochondrial health at the cellular level. The significance of comprehending the cellular and molecular principles of mitochondrial function is underscored by the association between metabolic and age-related diseases and mitochondrial malfunction.

In conclusion, mitochondria play a critical role in health and vitality. They influence numerous physiological processes in addition to energy production. Regaining and sustaining health and vigor require an understanding of the fundamental science underlying mitochondria and energy production.

This highlights the importance of mitochondria in energy production and general well-being, offering a thorough grasp of their function in health and vitality. The traditional function of mitochondria in oxidative phosphorylation, the significance of a well-balanced diet and micronutrient intake, and the evaluation of mitochondrial health through the use of high-content imaging technologies are all covered in the content.

Chapter Two

Mitochondrial Dysfunction and Health

A disorder known as mitochondrial dysfunction happens when the mitochondria are unable to generate enough energy to meet the body's requirements. Numerous health issues, such as chronic weariness, physical weakness, and cognitive impairment, can result from this illness. Numerous variables, such as genetic mutations, chemicals found in the environment, and lifestyle choices like poor eating, inactivity, and prolonged stress, have been related to mitochondrial dysfunction.

Monitoring variables like membrane potential, shape, and the buildup of reactive oxygen species (ROS) is part of evaluating the health of the mitochondria. Fluorescent dyes and high-content imaging techniques are used to assess mitochondrial health at the cellular level. Furthermore, it has been demonstrated that a variety of natural supplements, such as vitamins, minerals, and antioxidants, enhance mitochondrial health and maintain mitochondrial function.

To keep mitochondria functioning at their best, they must be nurtured and fed, which includes eating a diet rich in whole foods that is well-balanced. Omega-3 fatty acids, bone broth, and a high-fiber diet can promote mitochondrial health and guard against mitochondrial dysfunction. Because it encourages mitochondrial biogenesis, the process by which new mitochondria are created, exercise is also crucial for preserving healthy mitochondria.

Mitochondrial dysfunction is a disorder that can cause a number of health issues, such as persistent fatigue, weakened muscles, and cognitive loss. Monitoring variables like membrane potential, shape, and the buildup of reactive oxygen species (ROS) is part of evaluating the health of the mitochondria. Enhancing mitochondrial health and function can be achieved by taking natural supplements, exercising frequently, and eating a well-balanced, whole-foods-based diet.

This shed light on the factors that contribute to mitochondrial dysfunction, the techniques for evaluating the health of the mitochondria, and the natural supplements that can help the mitochondria function. The text highlights the significance of a healthy, whole-foods-based diet, regular exercise, and stress reduction in preserving mitochondrial health and averting mitochondrial malfunction.

- **Link between mitochondrial dysfunction and fatigue**

It is commonly known that fatigue and mitochondrial dysfunction are related. Because of their crucial role in energy production, mitochondria can malfunction and cause symptoms like weakness and exhaustion, among other health issues. One of the main signs of mitochondrial illness is fatigue, which is commonly defined as low energy, physical or mental exhaustion, decreased endurance, and the requirement for a protracted recuperation period following physical activity.

Studies have indicated that individuals with healthy mitochondria are less likely to have symptoms like weariness that are typical of mitochondrial dysfunction. Moderate to severe fatigue can be caused by mitochondrial malfunction, which can result in a loss of total energy at the cellular level. This may be especially important for those with a number of medical diseases, such as diabetes, cancer, fibromyalgia, and major mental illnesses, including bipolar disorder and schizophrenia.

More people are becoming aware of the significance mitochondrial function plays in both health and sickness, especially in the past 20 years. Numerous health issues, such as exhaustion, weakness, metabolic strokes, seizures, cardiomyopathy, and developmental or cognitive problems, are linked to mitochondrial dysfunction.

In conclusion, weariness and mitochondrial dysfunction are related, and this is an important part of general health and vitality. The significance of mitochondria in energy generation and their influence on a range of health disorders highlight the necessity of comprehending and managing mitochondrial malfunction in order to reduce fatigue and enhance general health.

- Diagnosis and treatment approaches

Diagnosis

It can be difficult to diagnose mitochondrial illness, and imaging investigations, genetic testing, and clinical examination are frequently needed. Mutations in nuclear or mitochondrial DNA that may be causing the illness can be found through genetic testing. MRIs and other imaging tests can be used to find structural anomalies in the brain or other organs that might be a sign of mitochondrial disease.

Making the right diagnosis of mitochondrial disease is crucial to choosing the right course of action. The goals of treating mitochondrial illness are to preserve optimum health, reduce symptoms with preventive treatments, and delay the disease's progression. The majority of professionals combine vitamins, improve overall health and nutrition, and stop symptoms from getting worse during illness and physiological stress. The symptoms of mitochondrial disease can also be managed with the aid of natural supplements, lifestyle changes, and emerging therapies.

A combination of imaging investigations, genetic testing, and clinical evaluation is used to diagnose mitochondrial illness. Maintaining optimum health, reducing symptoms through preventative measures, and delaying the disease's course are the major goals of treatment. The symptoms of mitochondrial illness can also be managed with the aid of natural supplements, lifestyle changes, and emerging medicines.

Treatment

The use of vitamins, improving overall health and nutrition, and taking preventative steps to lessen symptoms during illness and physiological stress are some of the treatment modalities for mitochondrial disease. For mitochondrial illness, several new treatments and lifestyle changes include:

Gene therapy: The goal of this strategy is to fix genetic alterations that cause mitochondrial disease.

Additionally, a novel and exciting strategy for treating mitochondrial disorders is gene therapy. In order to address the underlying cause of the disease, genetic material is introduced into the patient's cells and corrected or replaced as needed. Gene therapy has the potential to offer a permanent solution for mitochondrial disorders by treating the genetic abnormalities that are frequently caused by mutations in either the nuclear or mitochondrial DNA.

Because gene therapy for mitochondrial illnesses may be customized for each patient based on their unique genetic variants, age, sex, disease stage, and affected tissues, it is regarded as a precision medicine approach. This tailored approach may result in more focused and efficient treatment, possibly providing a permanent remedy for mitochondrial disease.

Even though gene therapy has great potential, there are issues and concerns that must be resolved before it can be successfully used to treat disorders of the mitochondria. The majority of mitochondrial illnesses are multi-systemic syndromes that impact several organs and may necessitate the therapeutic vector's extensive gene expression. Furthermore, the swift advancement of genome-editing technologies, like CRISPR/Cas9, presents the potential for accurately correcting undesirable mutations; however, hurdles associated with specific facets of mitochondrial biology must still be surmounted to ensure the successful implementation of gene therapy in mitochondrial disorders.

To sum up, gene therapy is a potentially effective and customized method for treating disorders related to mitochondria. Although there are obstacles and factors to take into account, gene therapy is a field of active study and development due to its potential to offer a permanent solution for mitochondrial illnesses.

Mitochondrial transplantation and transfer: In these procedures, a patient with a mitochondrial disease receives mitochondria from a healthy donor.

Moreover, mitochondrial illnesses can be treated with potential treatment strategies such as mitochondrial transplantation and transfer. In order to give a patient with a mitochondrial illness functional mitochondria for their cells, these techniques entail transferring healthy mitochondria from a donor to the patient. The salient features of these therapeutic modalities are as follows:

1. Mitochondrial transfer: Under healthy or pathological conditions, this process entails the intercellular transfer of mitochondria across cells. This behavior has been documented by researchers in both in vitro and in vivo experiments, indicating possible therapeutic uses.

2. Mitochondrial transplantation: Using isolated, functional mitochondria, this technique attempts to restore mitochondrial dysfunction. Heart ischemia can be effectively treated with mitochondrial transplantation, according to human clinical studies. Nonetheless, there are still issues with the immune response, the best dosage, the delivery method, the viability, the activity, and the maintenance of isolated mitochondria.

3. Optimal dosage and delivery method: For mitochondrial transplantation and transfer to be widely used as therapeutic procedures, standardized techniques must be developed. To guarantee the security and effectiveness of these therapies, researchers are attempting to optimize these parameters.

4. Feasibility and safety: The therapeutic benefits of mitochondrial transfer and transplantation on illnesses are still being investigated, and a broad acceptance of these treatments is constrained by their uncertain mechanism and efficacy. For mitochondrial transplantation and transfer to be successfully used in the treatment of mitochondrial disorders, several issues must be resolved.

To sum up, mitochondrial illnesses can be treated with potential treatment techniques such as mitochondrial transplantation and transfer. To address the issues surrounding these medicines' widespread adoption, researchers are focusing on maximizing the safe, effective dosage and delivery method.

Targeted genome editing: With this technique, mutations in mitochondrial DNA can be precisely corrected.

Additionally, targeted genome editing is a newly developed treatment strategy for disorders involving the mitochondria, especially those brought on by abnormalities in nuclear or mitochondrial DNA. Using genome-editing technologies like the CRISPR-Cas9 system, this method accurately fixes undesirable mutations and restores mitochondrial function.

Targeted genome editing in mitochondrial diseases has several important features, such as:

1. Precise repair of mutations: Unwanted mutations in the nuclear or mitochondrial DNA, which can result in mitochondrial disorders, can be precisely repaired using the CRISPR-Cas9 system.
2. Personalized strategy: Mitochondrial illnesses can be customized for each patient depending on their unique genetic variants, age, sex, disease stage, and the affected tissues. These syndromes are frequently multi-systemic and impact multiple organs.
3. Overcoming challenges: Improving the activity and broadening the target range of gene-editing technologies, as well as the effective delivery of guide RNA and Cas9

enzyme complexes into the mitochondria, are ongoing concerns and challenges.

To sum up, targeted genome editing is a very promising treatment strategy for disorders related to the mitochondria. This concept seeks to precisely correct mutations and restore mitochondrial function by utilizing cutting-edge gene-editing technology, providing patients with mitochondrial illnesses with a customized and successful treatment plan.

Diet and exercise: Maintaining mitochondrial function and enhancing general health can be achieved by eating a well-balanced, whole-foods diet and exercising on a regular basis.
More so, the management of mitochondrial illnesses greatly depends on diet and exercise. It has been demonstrated that these methods improve general health and mitochondrial function. Using the sources as a guide, the following are some salient points:

1. Nutritional Interventions: For people with mitochondrial illnesses, a healthy diet is crucial. It has been demonstrated that improving the

quantity and quality of calories enhances mitochondrial health. Although particular dietary modifications or limitations are not always advised, mitochondrial function can be supported by a comprehensive nutritional plan customized to each individual's needs.

2. Interventions Based on Exercise: It has been demonstrated that exercise increases the proportion of healthy, nonmutated mitochondrial DNA, lowers the burden of diseased mitochondria, and enhances muscular function and endurance. Frequent exercise can improve general health and well-being and is a crucial part of treatment for mitochondrial diseases.

3. Therapeutic Objectives: Increasing energy production or, at the very least, stabilizing disease signs and symptoms are the current therapeutic objectives for mitochondrial disease therapy. In order to accomplish these aims, diet and exercise are essential.

Dietary and exercise-based therapies are important parts of the strategy used to treat disorders involving the mitochondria. Regular exercise and a well-balanced diet can enhance general health, promote mitochondrial function, and help control the symptoms of mitochondrial illness.

Natural supplements: Studies have demonstrated the support and enhancement of mitochondrial function and health by supplements including Coenzyme Q10 (CoQ10), Alpha-lipoic Acid (ALA), L-Carnitine, NADH, and B vitamins.

Additionally, natural supplements can be very helpful in promoting mitochondrial health and reducing the signs and symptoms of illnesses related to the mitochondria. The following are some of the best natural supplements for enhancing mitochondrial function:

1. Coenzyme Q10 (CoQ10): Research has demonstrated that CoQ10, a nutrient that is essential for the synthesis of energy in cells, can improve the health of the mitochondria in people who have disorders related to the mitochondria.

2. Alpha-lipoic acid (ALA): Research has demonstrated that ALA, an antioxidant, can enhance mitochondrial activity in patients with mitochondrial disorders and help shield them from oxidative damage.

3. L-Carnitine: Research has demonstrated that the amino acid L-Carnitine supports the health of the mitochondria and lowers the chance of developing mitochondrial diseases.

4. NADH: Research has demonstrated that supplementing persons with mitochondrial illnesses with NADH, a coenzyme involved in energy production, can enhance their mitochondrial function.

5. B vitamins: Patients with mitochondrial illnesses have benefited from the use of B vitamins, especially thiamine and riboflavin, which have been shown to support mitochondrial activity and address energy impairment.

6. Resveratrol and ECGC-green tea extract: Studies have demonstrated that these

substances enhance the sirtuin pathways, which are beneficial to mitochondrial health and function.

7. Creatine: Though its efficacy has not yet been thoroughly investigated, creatine has been recommended as a pro-mitochondrial health supplement.

Before beginning any new supplement regimen, it is imperative to speak with a healthcare provider because every person's needs and health situations are unique.

Finally, a mix of pharmaceutical interventions, dietary changes, and novel therapies are used to treat mitochondrial dysfunction. These strategies seek to preserve optimum health, reduce symptoms, and impede the disease's advancement.

Chapter Three

Reclaiming Your Vitality

It takes a comprehensive approach to restore your vitality, involving your physical, mental, and emotional health. It entails taking a diverse approach to maintaining and improving vigor, vitality, and the general quality of life. The following are some salient points from the mentioned sources:

1. Physical Activity and Nature: Getting regular exercise and spending time in nature can help you feel more energized and have a fresh outlook. With its capacity to inspire contemplation and a change in perspective, nature is a wellspring of creativity and renewal.

2. Self-Care and Reflection: Self-care techniques like journaling, meditation, and goal-setting are frequently necessary for regaining vigor. Frequent introspection and self-evaluation can be helpful in identifying potential sources of vitality depletion and in formulating solutions.

3. Mindful Living: Maintaining and improving vitality can be greatly aided by cultivating a mindful and balanced lifestyle that includes a healthy diet, consistent exercise, and a dedication to lifelong learning.

4. Personal Growth and Creativity: Maintaining vitality may require embracing personal growth, creativity, and a dedication to lifelong learning. Taking part in creative and personal development activities can support the upkeep of motivation and purpose.

In conclusion, recovering vitality necessitates a whole strategy that includes exercise, self-care, mindful living, and personal development. Through the incorporation of these components into their everyday routines, people can strive to maintain and improve their general vitality and health.

- Strategies for overcoming mitochondrial fatigue

One typical indicator of mitochondrial disorders is mitochondrial tiredness, which has a serious negative effect on a person's quality of life. The following methods for overcoming mitochondrial tiredness are derived from the references given:

1. Natural Supplements: Studies have demonstrated that natural supplements with properties that enhance mitochondrial function and lessen fatigue in people with mitochondrial illnesses include Coenzyme Q10 (CoQ10), Alpha-lipoic Acid (ALA), L-Carnitine, NADH, and B vitamins.

2. Exercise: For people with mitochondrial disorders, regular exercise can help enhance mitochondrial function and lessen fatigue. It has been demonstrated that exercise increases the proportion of healthy, nonmutated mitochondrial DNA, lowers the burden of

diseased mitochondria, and enhances muscular function and endurance.

3. Nutrition: People with mitochondrial illnesses may experience less fatigue by eating a well-balanced, whole-foods diet, which supports mitochondrial function. While creatine monohydrate has offered an alternate energy source, nutritional therapies such as coenzyme Q10, idebenone, and triacylglycerol have been demonstrated to circumvent compromised respiratory enzymes or scavenge free radicals.

4. Avoiding Mitochondrial Dysfunction: You can lessen fatigue and prevent mitochondrial dysfunction by controlling stress, avoiding environmental pollutants, and getting enough sleep.

To sum up, there are several efficient ways to overcome mitochondrial fatigue, including natural supplements, exercise, a proper diet, and avoiding mitochondrial malfunction. These methods help maintain healthy mitochondria, enhance general well-being, and lessen the signs and symptoms of mitochondrial disorders.

- Functional medicine approach to vitality

A comprehensive and individualized strategy for resolving mitochondrial dysfunction and enhancing general health and well-being is part of a functional medicine approach to vitality. The following are some salient points from the mentioned sources:

Mitochondrial malfunction: A person's quality of life can be greatly impacted by mitochondrial malfunction, which is a prevalent underlying cause of many chronic diseases. Finding and treating the underlying causes of mitochondrial dysfunction, such as stress, dietary deficits, and environmental pollutants, is a key component of a functional medicine approach to vitality.

Nutrition: People with mitochondrial illnesses must follow a whole-food, well-balanced diet. A thorough diet regimen customized for each person can enhance mitochondrial function and enhance general health.

Exercise: People with mitochondrial illnesses may benefit from regular physical activity as it can help lower fatigue and enhance mitochondrial function. It has been demonstrated that exercise increases the proportion of healthy, nonmutated mitochondrial DNA, lowers the burden of diseased mitochondria, and enhances muscular function and endurance.

Natural Supplements: Studies have demonstrated that natural supplements with properties that enhance mitochondrial function and lessen fatigue in people with mitochondrial illnesses include Coenzyme Q10 (CoQ10), Alpha-lipoic Acid (ALA), L-Carnitine, NADH, and B vitamins.

Tailored Treatment: A tailored treatment plan that takes into account each person's particular needs and health concerns is a key component of the functional medicine approach to vitality. Combining dietary changes, complementary and alternative medicine, and cutting-edge treatments like gene therapy, mitochondrial transplantation and transfer, and targeted genome editing may be part of this strategy.

To sum up, a functional medicine approach to vitality entails treating mitochondrial dysfunction in a thorough and individualized manner in order to enhance general health and wellbeing. Personalized treatment regimens, natural supplements, exercise, and proper nutrition can all help to improve mitochondrial function and lessen the symptoms of mitochondrial illnesses.

Chapter Four

The Power of Mitochondria in Health Restoration

The ability of mitochondria to restore health is a vital component of overall wellbeing. Often referred to as the "powerhouse of the cell," mitochondria are key for producing adenosine triphosphate (ATP), an energy source necessary for the health and function of cells. Understanding the role of mitochondria in health and disease is essential for designing ways to support their function and enhance overall wellness. Mitochondrial malfunction has been connected to a number of health issues.

It has been established that mitochondria are the main source of ATP, accounting for more than 90% of the energy needed for cell metabolism. They are necessary for preserving regular and healthy cellular functions since they are also engaged in other facets of cell metabolism and function. Nonetheless, a number of human diseases have been linked to mitochondrial dysfunction, emphasizing how important it is to comprehend and treat problems pertaining to mitochondrial health.

A thorough and individualized plan is used in a functional medicine approach to vitality to address mitochondrial dysfunction and enhance general health. The core reasons for mitochondrial dysfunction, such as stress, dietary shortages, and environmental pollutants, must be found and addressed as part of this strategy. Furthermore, studies have demonstrated that a healthy, whole-foods-based diet, consistent exercise, and the use of natural supplements can enhance mitochondrial function and lessen fatigue in those with mitochondrial illnesses.

To sum up, the ability of mitochondria to restore health is a vital component in fostering general well-being. A person's vitality, energy, and general health can be enhanced by learning about the role mitochondria play in health and disease and putting strategies in place to support their function.

- **Mitochondria and their impact on overall well-being**

Beyond just producing energy, mitochondria are essential to both health and sickness. They do this through a variety of processes. Numerous illnesses, such as the metabolic syndrome, neurological disorders, cancer, infectious and cardiovascular diseases, and inflammatory disorders, have all been related to mitochondrial dysfunction. Thus, maintaining mitochondrial function is essential for general health and vigor.

When it comes to vitality, a functional medicine method employs a thorough, holistic, and root-cause-focused approach to treating chronic illness and restoring health. The core reasons for mitochondrial dysfunction, such as stress, dietary shortages, and environmental pollutants, must be found and addressed as part of this strategy. Furthermore, studies have demonstrated that a healthy, whole-foods-based diet, consistent exercise, and the use of natural supplements can enhance mitochondrial function and lessen fatigue in those with mitochondrial illnesses.

One of the few strategies that has been shown to increase mitochondrial functioning and reduce the number of dysfunctional mitochondria is exercise. It has been demonstrated to enhance muscle function and endurance while lowering the burden of sick mitochondria and raising the proportion of healthy, non mutated mitochondrial DNA. The present objectives of treatment for mitochondrial diseases are to enhance energy production or maintain illness signs and symptoms at a minimum.

To sum up, energy, concentration, vitality, and metabolism all depend on the maintenance and nourishment of mitochondria. To restore health and treat patients with chronic illnesses, an all-encompassing, integrative strategy that focuses on the underlying causes of the condition is essential. This approach should include natural supplements, exercise, and proper nutrition. Through the management of mitochondrial health, people can strive to enhance their general well-being, vigor, and energy.

- Potential for vitality restoration through mitochondrial health

Mitochondria are essential for general health since they affect many other processes in addition to energy production. Numerous health issues, such as metabolic syndrome, neurological disorders, cancer, infectious and cardiovascular illnesses, and inflammatory disorders, have all been connected to mitochondrial dysfunction. Thus, maintaining mitochondrial function is essential for general health and vigor.

An integrative, holistic, and root-cause-focused approach is employed in functional medicine to treat chronic disease patients and restore health. The core reasons for mitochondrial dysfunction, such as stress, dietary shortages, and environmental pollutants, must be found and addressed as part of this strategy. Furthermore, studies have demonstrated that a whole-foods-based, well-balanced diet, consistent exercise, and the use of natural supplements can promote mitochondrial function and lessen fatigue in people with mitochondrial diseases.

Mitochondrial transplantation and transfer, which involve utilizing isolated working mitochondria to recover mitochondrial malfunction, are promising treatment methods for disorders involving the mitochondria. These applications have been proven to be beneficial in the treatment of myocardial ischemia and other mitochondrial diseases, and they have the potential to treat abnormalities of the mitochondria.

In conclusion, a promising topic of study in the fields of functional medicine and mitochondrial illnesses is the possibility of vitality restoration through mitochondrial health. To address mitochondrial dysfunction and enhance general health and vitality, viable therapeutic approaches include mitochondrial transplantation and transfer, as well as a comprehensive functional medicine approach. Through the management of mitochondrial health, people can strive to enhance their general well-being, vigor, and energy.

Chapter Five

Your Ultimate Vitality Pharmacy

The phrase "Your Ultimate Vitality Pharmacy" refers to a holistic strategy that uses nutrients, botanicals, nutraceuticals, and other substances to support health and vitality. "Ultimate Vitality" by Innovative Wellness Inc., a concoction of nutrients, nutraceuticals, botanicals, and Krebs cycle intermediates intended to promote effective mitochondrial function, is one particular product that fits with this idea.

The phrase "ultimate vitality pharmacy" refers to the employment of different interventions to improve general well-being and mitochondrial function in the context of mitochondrial health. This could involve making lifestyle changes, taking certain supplements, and trying out new treatments that target mitochondrial malfunction and enhance mitochondrial health.

Exercise has been demonstrated in studies to enhance mitochondrial activity and lessen the load of unhealthy mitochondria. Furthermore, some supplements might function as substitute energy sources or get around metabolic obstacles inside the mitochondria, which might make them useful for treating some clinical symptoms and delaying the course of some diseases.

Additionally, treating the underlying causes of mitochondrial dysfunction and implementing a variety of interventions—such as vitamin use, nutrition optimization, and preventing symptom aggravation during illness and physiological stress—are all part of a functional medicine approach to mitochondrial dysfunction.

To sum up, the idea behind "Your Ultimate Vitality Pharmacy" is a holistic strategy for promoting health and vitality, especially when it comes to mitochondrial health. This could entail using certain formulations, changing one's lifestyle, and utilizing cutting-edge treatments meant to enhance mitochondrial health and well-being in general.

- Medications and supplements for vitality

Many times, a multimodal strategy is used to treat mitochondrial illnesses, involving the use of vitamins and pharmaceuticals. It's crucial to remember that there isn't a known medication treatment for mitochondrial illnesses at this time. Rather, the emphasis is on symptom management and enhancing general health and wellbeing.

1. Nutritional Interventions: Energy impairment and its aftereffects have been the focus of numerous nutritionally based therapy approaches. For example, it has been demonstrated that coenzyme Q10, idebenone, and triacylglycerol can scavenge free radicals and circumvent faulty respiratory enzymes,

while creatine monohydrate offers an alternate energy source.

2. Therapies Based on Exercise: One of the few strategies that has been shown to increase mitochondrial functioning and reduce the number of dysfunctional mitochondria is exercise. It has been demonstrated to enhance muscular function and endurance, decrease the burden of diseased mitochondria, and raise the proportion of healthy, non mutated mitochondrial DNA.

3. Approach to Functional Medicine: When treating patients with chronic illnesses, a functional medicine approach to mitochondrial dysfunction focuses on treating the underlying cause of the illness and restoring health in a thorough and integrated manner. The core reasons for mitochondrial dysfunction, such as stress, dietary shortages, and environmental pollutants, must be found and addressed as part of this strategy.

4. Supplements: Although there isn't a known medication to treat mitochondrial illnesses, several supplements have been tried to reduce some clinical symptoms and may be able to slow down the disease's progression. It's crucial to remember that there is a dearth of high-caliber scientific evidence to support the use of these medicines, and their efficacy is currently being debated.

In conclusion, dietary interventions, exercise-based therapies, and a functional medicine approach are all used in the current therapy of mitochondrial illnesses in order to address the underlying reasons for mitochondrial malfunction. As of right now, there is no approved medication treatment for mitochondrial illnesses; however, several supplements have been utilized to address energy limitation and its aftereffects.

- Harnessing the body's life force for health restoration

Using the life force of the body to restore health means maximizing mitochondrial function, which is critical for general health and vigor. A vital component of energy production, mitochondria also influence other processes in addition to energy production. Numerous health issues, such as metabolic syndrome, neurological disorders, cancer, infectious and cardiovascular illnesses, and inflammatory disorders, have all been connected to mitochondrial dysfunction.

An integrative, holistic, and root-cause-focused approach is employed in functional medicine to treat chronic disease patients and restore health. The core reasons for mitochondrial dysfunction, such as stress, dietary shortages, and environmental pollutants, must be found and addressed as part of this strategy. Furthermore, studies have demonstrated that a whole-foods-based, well-balanced diet, consistent exercise, and the use of natural supplements can enhance mitochondrial function and lessen fatigue in people with mitochondrial diseases.

Optimizing mitochondrial activity is the key to utilizing the body's life energy. This can be accomplished by a variety of interventions, such as exercise, diet, and natural supplements. One of the few strategies that has been shown to increase mitochondrial functioning and reduce the number of diseased mitochondria is exercise. Furthermore, some supplements might function as substitute energy sources or get around metabolic obstacles inside the mitochondria, which might make them useful for treating some clinical symptoms and delaying the course of some diseases.

To sum up, the key to restoring health and improving the body's life force is to maximize mitochondrial activity, which is critical for general health and vitality. To restore health and treat patients with chronic illnesses, an all-encompassing, integrative strategy that focuses on the underlying causes of the condition is essential. This approach should include natural supplements, exercise, and proper nutrition. Through the management of mitochondrial health, people can strive to enhance their general well-being, vigor, and energy.

Chapter Six

Regenerating Health with Mitochondria

Utilizing mitochondria to boost general health and energy is known as "regenerating health with mitochondria." Beyond their role in energy production, mitochondria have a multitude of other functions that are important for both health and sickness. Numerous health issues, such as metabolic syndrome, neurological disorders, cancer, infectious and cardiovascular illnesses, and inflammatory disorders, have all been connected to mitochondrial dysfunction.

When it comes to vitality, a functional medicine method employs a thorough, holistic, and root-cause-focused approach to treating chronic illness and restoring health. The core reasons for mitochondrial dysfunction, such as stress, dietary shortages, and environmental pollutants, must be found and addressed as part of this strategy. Furthermore, studies have demonstrated that a healthy, whole-foods-based diet, consistent exercise, and the use of natural supplements can enhance mitochondrial function and lessen fatigue in those with mitochondrial illnesses.

Using the potential of mitochondria to restore health can be accomplished by a number of strategies, such as:

Exercise: One of the few scientifically supported strategies for enhancing mitochondrial function and lowering the load of dysfunctional mitochondria is exercise. It has been demonstrated to enhance muscle function and endurance while lowering the burden of sick mitochondria and raising the proportion of healthy, nonmutated mitochondrial DNA.

Nutrition: People with mitochondrial illnesses must follow a whole-food, well-balanced diet. Overall health can be enhanced and mitochondrial function supported with a personalized, all-inclusive diet plan.

<u>*Natural Supplements*</u>: Studies on people with mitochondrial disorders have demonstrated that using natural supplements including coenzyme Q10 (CoQ10), ALA, L-carnitine, NADH, and B vitamins can improve mitochondrial function and lessen fatigue.

<u>*Mitochondrial Transplantation and Transfer*</u>: Using isolated, functional mitochondria, mitochondrial dysfunction can be recovered through mitochondrial transplantation and transfer, two potentially effective treatment strategies for disorders involving the mitochondria. These applications have been found to be beneficial in the treatment of myocardial ischemia and other mitochondrial diseases, and they have the potential to treat other ailments of the mitochondria.

In conclusion, using mitochondria to regenerate health entails utilizing their potential to enhance general health and vigor. To restore health and cure patients with chronic illnesses, an all-encompassing, integrative strategy that addresses the underlying causes of the disease and includes natural supplements, exercise, nutrition, and cutting-edge therapies like mitochondrial transplantation and transfer is essential.

- Organ regeneration and its connection to mitochondrial health

Beyond their role in producing energy, mitochondria are involved in many different processes that affect both health and disease. The production of new mitochondria and striking a balance for the health of the mitochondria depend on mitochondrial function. Mitophagy, mitochondrial biogenesis, and mitochondrial microRNAs all play significant roles in tissue regeneration by influencing ATP synthesis, ROS generation, and mitochondrial metabolism. An all-encompassing, integrative approach that focuses on treating the underlying causes of chronic diseases and restoring mitochondrial functioning can be found in the use of physiological stress, which promotes tolerance to stressors, adaptability, and resistance. It is commonly known that mitochondria play a key role in energy metabolism, signal transduction, and aging in post-mitotic tissues. There is growing evidence that stem cell rejuvenation and aging are influenced by mitochondrial activity and that mitochondrial-linked signaling plays a critical role in stem cell function. Therefore, vitality, tissue regeneration, and general well-being depend on optimizing mitochondrial health.

- Mitochondria and the possibility of disease elimination

The function of mitochondria in health and illness is multifaceted and goes beyond simple energy production. Numerous health issues, such as metabolic syndrome, neurological disorders, cancer, infectious and cardiovascular illnesses, and inflammatory disorders, have all been connected to mitochondrial dysfunction. According to "The Mitochondrial Miracle: Reclaiming Your Health and Vitality," people with chronic illnesses can regain their health and be treated with an integrative, holistic approach that focuses on the underlying causes of their illness.

It is commonly known that mitochondria play a crucial role in the generation of energy, signal transmission, and aging of post-mitotic tissues. The production of new mitochondria and striking a balance for the health of the mitochondria depend on mitochondrial function. Mitophagy, mitochondrial biogenesis, and mitochondrial microRNAs all play significant roles in tissue regeneration by influencing ATP synthesis, ROS generation, and mitochondrial metabolism.

An all-encompassing, integrative approach that focuses on treating the underlying causes of chronic diseases and restoring mitochondrial functioning can be found in the use of physiological stress, which promotes tolerance to stressors, adaptability, and resistance. The ensuing tactics have the capacity to eradicate illnesses and enhance mitochondrial health: Exercise, Nutrition, Natural Supplements, Mitochondrial Transplantation, and Transfer. Mitochondria are important for both health and disease, and maximizing their activity is critical for life, the healing of damaged tissue, and general wellbeing. People can improve their vitality, energy, and general well-being by taking care of their mitochondrial health, which may also help to prevent diseases associated with mitochondrial malfunction.

Chapter Seven

The Wondrous WNT Pathway: The Ultimate Fountain of Youth?

Development, differentiation, and homeostatic renewal are just a few of the cellular functions that the WNT (Wingless N-Cadherin) pathway is essential for. Numerous medical illnesses, including cancer, metabolic diseases, and neurological disorders, have been linked to it. The WNT pathway is called "The Ultimate Fountain of Youth" in "The Mitochondrial Miracle: Reclaiming Your Health and Vitality" because of its capacity to encourage renewal and fend off degenerative diseases.

The following processes are significantly impacted by the WNT pathway:

Stem Cell Function: To promote tissue regeneration and repair, progenitor and stem cell balance must be maintained, which is accomplished by the WNT pathway. It may be possible to slow down the aging process and enhance both health and disease by modifying WNT signaling.

Liver Development and Regeneration: A crucial regulator of liver development, differentiation, and homeostatic renewal is the classical WNT pathway. It has been demonstrated to be involved in liver regeneration and may be used as a target for liver diseases.

Metabolic disorders and cancer: Diverse forms of metabolic disorders and cancer have been linked to aberrant WNT signaling. The development of treatment plans for various illnesses may benefit from focusing on the WNT pathway.

Neurodegenerative Disorders: Alzheimer's and Parkinson's illnesses, among others, have been linked to the pathophysiology of the WNT pathway. Treatment for these illnesses may benefit from WNT signaling modulation.

Targeting the WNT pathway may provide advantages, but there are drawbacks and uncertainties about its effectiveness and safety. The WNT signaling cascade is a desirable target for more study and the creation of therapeutic approaches due to its complexity and the possible hazards connected with its manipulation.

To sum up, the WNT pathway has the ability to prevent degenerative diseases and promote rejuvenation, making it "the ultimate fountain of youth" with immense promise. To completely understand the WNT pathway's involvement in health and disease and to develop safe and effective therapeutic options, further research is necessary; thus, it is important to take into account the risks and challenges of targeting it.

- Exploring the WNT pathway for health and vitality

The possible effects of the WNT (Wingless N-Cadherin) pathway on vigor and health have drawn attention, especially when it comes to pluripotent stem cells' cell cycle and mitochondrial dynamics. Recent research has shown connections between the pathways governing the cell cycle and mitochondrial dynamics, indicating that modifications in the intrinsic regulation of mitochondrial dynamics, which in turn impacts the final fate of the cell, are influenced by Wnt signaling activity.

Moreover, the WNT pathway has been linked to neuroprotection, as evidenced by its capacity to stop mitochondrial membrane permeabilization, protecting against neurodegeneration. Furthermore, research on the impact of Wnt signaling regulation by mitochondria on carcinogenesis has shown a two-way communication between mitochondria and the Wnt pathway. This creates a feedforward loop whereby Wnt activation drives mitochondrial regulation and vice versa.

There has been discussion over the WNT pathway's potential as "The Ultimate Fountain of Youth" and how it affects the body's renewal and prevents degenerative disorders. Targeting and modulating the WNT pathway has the potential to promote healing, rejuvenation, and the eradication of illnesses, which is why it is a focal area for innovative medical interventions and scientific discoveries.

The significance of the canonical WNT pathway in tissue and organ regeneration is further highlighted by the identification of this pathway as a critical regulator in liver development, differentiation, and homeostatic renewal. It is anticipated that improving our knowledge of this route will help with drug screening, disease modeling, and the creation of tissue and organ substitutes for regenerative medicine.

In conclusion, the WNT pathway is important for maintaining health, vitality, and preventing disease because of its possible effects on neuroprotection, carcinogenesis, mitochondrial and cell cycle dynamics, and liver formation and regeneration. Although more investigation is necessary to completely understand its intricacies and its uses, the WNT pathway is an intriguing field of study in the pursuit of health and vitality.

- **Preventing degenerative diseases through scientific breakthroughs**

By applying state-of-the-art research and technology to create novel treatments and therapies, scientists can prevent degenerative diseases. Millions of individuals worldwide suffer from degenerative diseases, which include cancer, Parkinson's, and Alzheimer's. These illnesses are long-lasting and progress slowly. Even if the preventive measures in place are beneficial, new methods for controlling and preventing these diseases must be developed through medical research.

Research on stem cells is one field where scientific advances could revolutionize the study of Parkinson's and other late-onset diseases. There is an endless supply of material for research because scientists can reprogram a patient's skin cells to become brain or liver cells. This method could be a more successful way to find novel medications to treat late-onset conditions like Alzheimer's, arthritis, and hearing loss, as it does not include the use of embryos.

The WNT pathway, which has been linked to neuroprotection and the possibility of avoiding degenerative disorders, is another field of scientific advancement. The WNT pathway is important for liver development and regeneration, cancer, metabolic disorders, and stem cell function. The development of treatment plans for various illnesses may benefit from focusing on the WNT pathway.

Another area where science has made strides in preventing degenerative diseases is nutrition. A thorough diet regimen customized for each person can enhance general health and boost mitochondrial function. In addition, lowering the pain threshold in multiple sclerosis can be achieved with a well-balanced, whole-foods diet combined with physical activity and aerobics.

In conclusion, using state-of-the-art research and technology to create novel treatments and cures is a key component in preventing degenerative diseases through scientific discoveries. Scientific advancements in the fields of nutrition, stem cell research, and the WNT pathway show promise in the prevention and management of degenerative disorders. Although additional investigation is required to properly comprehend these fields, they provide promising avenues for the creation of fresh strategies for the management and avoidance of degenerative illnesses.

Chapter Eight

The Power of Stem Cells

Because stem cells have the potential to revolutionize research into degenerative diseases like Alzheimer's, Parkinson's, and cancer, they have been the focus of scientific advances in "Reclaiming Your Health and Vitality" Because stem cells may develop into other types of cells, they hold great promise for the therapy of diseases and for regenerative medicine.

It is generally known that mitochondria are important for energy metabolism, signal transduction, and aging in post-mitotic tissues. They also play a critical role in stem cell destiny and aging. Numerous health issues, such as metabolic syndrome, neurological disorders, cancer, infectious and cardiovascular illnesses, and inflammatory disorders, have all been connected to mitochondrial dysfunction. Positively, a few in vitro investigations have shown that stem cells may replace damaged mitochondria with healthy ones in order to restore energy.

Further studies have shown that the activity of stem cells generally depends on mitochondrial dynamics and that the differentiation of different types of stem cells—such as those for blood and fat cells, and more recently, neurons—is aided by mitochondrial ROS signaling. Glycolysis, a cytoplasmic process that produces ATP, is the main energy-producing mechanism for stem cells as opposed to oxidative phosphorylation, which is a mitochondria-dependent activity that most mature, specialized cells prefer. In order to preserve the best possible learning and memory, researchers are trying to discover novel approaches to enhance mitochondrial function in stem cells through nutritional or pharmaceutical interventions.

In conclusion, stem cells show promise for advancing our understanding of degenerative disorders through the donation of functioning mitochondria to replace damaged ones and restore energy. Researchers are trying to identify novel strategies to enhance mitochondrial function in stem cells because it is crucial for stem cell function. These scientific discoveries could lead to the creation of fresh strategies for the management and avoidance of degenerative illnesses.

- Significance of stem cells in health and vitality

Because of their exceptional capacity for regeneration and their potential for use in the treatment of a wide range of illnesses, stem cells are extremely important for maintaining health and vitality. The following are some important facets of stem cell significance:

Tissue Regeneration: Stem cells are a promising treatment option for conditions including diabetes, heart disease, and spinal cord injuries because they have the ability to develop into multiple cell types and regenerate and mend tissue.

Disease Treatment: By substituting for cells lost due to illness or injury, stem cells provide new possibilities for treating diseases. For instance, stem cell treatment has been utilized to treat a variety of illnesses, including musculoskeletal conditions like osteoarthritis and neurological illnesses like Alzheimer's.

Drug Development and Testing: Researchers examining the onset and course of diseases can find value in stem cells as they can be utilized to evaluate novel medications and create model systems for comprehending illnesses.

Regenerative Medicine: By directing stem cells to become particular cells, they can be utilized in regenerative medicine to replace diseased cells with healthy ones.

Organ and Tissue Generation: Organ transplantation is becoming increasingly dependent on stem cell technology due to the capacity of stem cells to build new tissues and organs.

Even with stem cells' exciting potential, there is still a lot more research to be done in the lab and in the clinic before these cells may be used in therapeutic settings. Scholars are currently engaged in the development of novel techniques aimed at enhancing mitochondrial function in stem cells, comprehending the fundamental characteristics of stem cells, and isolating and culturing these cells for further therapeutic applications. The importance of stem cells to health and vitality is predicted to increase as scientific knowledge and methods improve, providing fresh hope for the treatment of several illnesses and the creation of novel therapies.

- Stem cells as the body's repair kit

Because they are essential to the body's regeneration and repair mechanisms, stem cells are important for preserving health and vigor. Because stem cells can differentiate into numerous cell types, they can replace old or damaged cells and aid in the rejuvenation of tissues and organs. This ability to develop into diverse cell types is a key factor in the role of stem cells in these processes. Treating age-related ailments and degenerative disorders may greatly benefit from this regenerative potential.

The significance of the relationship between mitochondrial activity and the preservation of stem cell vitality has been highlighted by recent studies on the role of mitochondria in stem cell destiny and aging. It has been demonstrated that mitochondrial dynamics are crucial for the function of stem cells and that the differentiation of different types of stem cells, such as those for blood, fat cells, and neurons, is greatly aided by mitochondrial ROS signaling. Moreover, promising in vitro research has shown that stem cells can replace damaged mitochondria with healthy ones, restoring cellular energy and providing a possible means of improving cellular resilience and function.

The potential therapeutic applications of stem cells provide more evidence of their significance for maintaining health and vitality. As a unique way to address mitochondrial malfunction and its related health consequences, stem cell-derived mitochondria transplantation has emerged as a promising therapy for neurological disorders such as mitochondrial encephalomyopathy. This novel approach has enormous potential to improve the field of regenerative medicine and lessen the effects of mitochondrial illnesses.

In conclusion, stem cells are essential to tissue regeneration, illness treatment, and regenerative medicine. They function as the body's repair kit. The importance of stem cells in preserving health and vitality is highlighted by their tight association with mitochondrial function and their capacity to donate healthy mitochondria. This opens up new possibilities for treating degenerative disorders and developing therapeutic interventions.

Conclusion

In conclusion, "The Mitochondrial Miracle: Reclaiming Your Health and Vitality" has examined the role that mitochondria play in preserving health and vitality as well as the possible benefits of several treatments for enhancing mitochondrial performance. The significance of comprehending the intricacies of mitochondrial function and its function in both health and sickness has been emphasized throughout the book. With an emphasis on an all-encompassing, integrative approach that addresses the underlying causes of health issues, the book provides insightful information and useful guidance to anybody looking to harness the power of mitochondria to enhance their health and well-being.

Key takeaways from the book include:

1. The critical role that mitochondria play in the synthesis of cellular energy, aging, and disease, as well as the possibility that a number of different health disorders are caused by mitochondrial malfunction.

2. The significance of treating environmental pollutants, dietary deficits, and stress as the primary drivers of mitochondrial dysfunction in order to reestablish health and vigor.

3. The ability of different therapies to support mitochondrial function and lessen fatigue in people with mitochondrial illnesses. These interventions include diet, exercise, and natural supplements.

4. The potential for scientific advances in mitochondrial health, including studies on stem cells, the WNT pathway, and novel treatments for disorders involving the mitochondria.

People may take charge of their health and vitality and use the power of mitochondria to reclaim their well-being and conquer the obstacles of contemporary life by comprehending the role of mitochondria in health and disease and putting the useful suggestions in the book into practice.

References

Pizzorno, J. (2016). The Mitochondrial Metabolic Therapy (MMT) Handbook. Integrative Medicine Publishing.

Wahls, T. (2014). Minding My Mitochondria 2nd Edition: How I overcame secondary progressive multiple sclerosis (MS) and got out of my wheelchair. Wahls Publishing.

Parikh, S., & Goldstein, A. (2013). A modern approach to the treatment of mitochondrial disease. Current treatment options in neurology, 15(4), 539-551.

Wallace, D. C. (2012). Mitochondria and cancer. Nature Reviews Cancer, 12(10), 685-698.

Lee, H. C., Wei, Y. H., & Mitochondrial DNA, W. G. (2005). Oxidative stress, mitochondrial DNA mutation, and apoptosis in aging.

Experimental Biology and Medicine, 230(9), 639-647.

Kowaltowski, A. J., & Vercesi, A. E. (1999). Mitochondrial damage induced by conditions of oxidative stress. Free Radical Biology and Medicine, 26(3-4), 463-471.

Wallace, D. C. (1999). Mitochondrial diseases in man and mouse. Science, 283(5407), 1482-1488.

Wallace, D. C. (1992). Mitochondrial genetics: a paradigm for aging and degenerative diseases?. Science, 256(5057), 628-632.

About the Author

With a steadfast commitment to healthcare spanning seven years, Dr. Nikolai J. Graham stands as a dedicated medical practitioner and a pioneering researcher specializing in rare genetic disorders. Driven by a passion for unraveling the complexities of genetic anomalies, Dr. Graham has become a beacon of expertise at the intersection of clinical practice and groundbreaking research.

As a seasoned medical practitioner, Dr. Graham has demonstrated unwavering dedication to providing compassionate and comprehensive care to patients facing rare genetic disorders. His seven years of clinical experience reflect a commitment to staying at the forefront of medical advancements, ensuring that each patient receives individualized attention and cutting-edge treatments tailored to their unique needs.

Beyond the clinic, Dr. Graham has emerged as a distinguished researcher in the realm of rare genetic disorders. His contributions to the scientific community include pioneering investigations into the underlying mechanisms of these conditions. By combining clinical insights with a fervor for discovery, Dr. Graham is actively engaged in advancing our understanding of rare genetic disorders, striving to unlock new avenues for diagnosis, treatment, and, ultimately, improved patient outcomes.

Recognizing the importance of raising awareness about rare genetic disorders, Dr. Nikolai J. Graham is not only a practitioner and researcher but also a vocal advocate and educator. Through various channels, he seeks to demystify these conditions, fostering a broader understanding among both the medical community and the public.

Dr. Graham's approach revolves around placing patients at the center of their healthcare journey. By blending clinical expertise with a compassionate bedside manner, he ensures that individuals facing rare genetic disorders receive not only top-tier medical care but also the support and understanding crucial for navigating the complexities of their conditions.

In the realm where medical practice and research intersect, Dr. Nikolai J. Graham stands as a beacon of hope, striving to illuminate the path toward improved treatments, enhanced diagnostics, and, ultimately, a brighter future for those affected by rare genetic disorders.